The Ideal food and nutrition for pregnancy:

The best approach to effective prenatal nutrition and lifestyle.

By

Helen V. Williamson

Table of contents

Introduction

Pregnancy is exciting; however, for most ladies, there are various difficulties they face going with financial and close-to-home stressors, hormone induced movements. Being well informed about pregnancy, as well as possible inconveniences and side effects, can help ease nervousness and help moms-to-be and their accomplices center around the supernatural occurrence of labor. They feel confident and ready as they enter their new jobs as guardians.

A parent is a fantastic choice. For some individuals, the fantasy about having a youngster can contrast extraordinarily with the truth. Pregnancy can be dumbfounding as the body goes through different changes to help the creating child. The pregnant lady's organization with her life partner can likewise develop during the pregnancy as guardians enter another period of their relationship.

Each pregnancy is unique; the side effects experienced rely upon the singular lady. Some

get the cover of pregnancy or obscured pigmentation on the face, while others don't—a few encounter morning infection and sickness. Pregnant ladies have different decisions in light of their convictions and requirements. For instance, the type of food varieties and supplements would cause their children to thrive. There's no exact decision to make concerning any choices related to conceiving an offspring and bringing up a youngster. Instead, when pregnant ladies look for data and medical services suppliers who can give dependable direction, they become better prepared to settle on appropriate decisions for themselves and their loved ones.
In this book, You will figure out All that you want to be familiar with consuming the proper nourishments, rehearsing a solid way of life for the well-being of you and your unborn kid and methods by which you can adapt to pregnancy stress.

Chapter 1

Why should I eat the Ideal food ?

Eating Sound During Pregnancy, For the most part, there are numerous advantages to practicing good eating habits. For example, a nutritious eating regimen yields a lady more maintainable energy, a more grounded, insusceptible framework, and a diminished gamble of infection. Pregnant ladies should be especially cautious about what they eat because they eat for their well-being. However, they are additionally eating for their child's well-being! When a lady eats well during her pregnancy, she diminishes the possibility of inconveniences, for example, iron deficiency, low birth weight, and birth surrenders. Eating great can likewise assist with disagreeable pregnancy side effects! The following are a few different advantages of a solid pregnancy diet.

Why is a healthy eating routine important for Mother And Child?

Less complication

it is difficult to fight of unhealthy pregnancy cravings; however, it is worth the effort over the long run for you and your child's well-being. If you're not practicing a proper eating routine, you could suffer from gestational diabetes, iron deficiency, urinary parcel contaminations, and your child being brought into the world with birth surrenders. Great nourishment during pregnancy can further develop work and conveyance, which is never terrible!.

Increased amount of energy

Sometimes regardless of what you do, fatigue is difficult to control - particularly in the early weeks with every one of the hormonal changes your body is going through. Keeping a healthy eating routine and eating each 3-4 hours will keep your energy up. It's memorable's Essential your iron utilization ought to be multiplied when you are pregnant to assist with supporting your expanded blood volume and advance iron stockpiling for the developing baby.

For effective Fetal development

A reasonable eating regimen is what your child needs to develop well. It would help if you targeted eating something like 300 additional calories daily than you ordinarily would. Be that as it may, you would instead not get carried away as it can prompt inconveniences like toxemia and gestational diabetes. However, nutrients and supplements that will warrant solid child incorporation are not restricted to folate or folic corrosive, L-ascorbic acid, vitamin A, calcium, fiber, foods grown from the ground, entire grains, and an adequate measure of protein and fat.

Improved sleep

various factors can keep you up around evening time during your pregnancy, for example, sickness, late-night washroom breaks, or a throbbing painfulness! Ensuring you are eating complete dinners every day, and avoiding an excessive amount of caffeine, will assist with your magnificence rest. The nutrients and necessary minerals during pregnancy, like vitamin B, calcium, and iron, help with rest.

Reduced chances of becoming ill

Pregnant ladies are more defenseless to specific contaminations like this season's virus.

A sound eating routine and rest can keep this from occurring. Albeit a little virus will, in all probability, not influence your child, experiencing pregnancy side effects is sufficiently terrible and being debilitated on top of that isn't engaging. Attempting to try not to become ill overall is a sure thing!

Chapter 2

The Ideal nutrient Intake during pregnancy

Next are supplements that are exceptionally advantageous to you and your child's well-being and improvement, and they incorporate.

Protein

Protein keeps up with muscle and body tissue. It is likewise key for a child's development - particularly during the second and third trimesters. Assuming you are a veggie-lover, you can meet your protein needs by eating food varieties that are finished protein sources. A total protein has all the fundamental "building blocks" (amino acids) your body needs. Every day, eat an assortment of protein sources to give your body essential amino acids. Veggie-lover protein choices include beans, milk, yogurt, eggs, and soy. Pregnant veggie lovers can meet their protein needs with soy, a complete protein source. Sources of soy protein include soy milk, cheddar, soy yogurt, tofu, and tempeh. Instances of other protein-rich veggie lover food varieties are nuts and beans (red kidney beans, chickpeas, dark beans, and so forth.).

Starches

Starches are an essential source of energy for the body. Natural products, vegetables, grains, and dairy items contain starches. Entire grains are a significant sources of supplements, like dietary fiber. They likewise give an assortment of medical advantages. Other significant starch food varieties incorporate advanced refined grains. These grains have the additional advantage of iron and folic corrosive, two fundamental supplements for the child's development. They include biscuits, yogurt, bagels, cereals, bread, and natural products. Other starch-containing decisions for dinners or tidbits incorporate saltines, bread, and pasta.

Fats

Fat is key for good nourishment, well-being, and the capacity for numerous significant

nutrients. Like starches and protein, dietary fat is a significant source of energy for the body. Certain food varieties that contain fat stockpile the body with fundamental unsaturated fats. Fundamental unsaturated fats will be fats the body doesn't make, so they should be remembered for the eating routine. In particular, fundamental unsaturated fats are basic for the child's development and advancement.
Sources of unsaturated fat incorporate fish, vegetable oils (canola, soybean, olive, nut, safflower, and sunflower oils), nuts, and flaxseeds. All ladies, including those pregnant or breastfeeding, should follow these suggestions.
DHA is an unsaturated fat significant for children's cerebrum and eye improvement. Slick fish, for example, salmon and fish, contain DHA.

Calcium

Calcium is significant for the development of solid bones and teeth. Calcium admission is fundamental for all ladies. Particularly pregnant ladies more youthful than 25 years of age whose bones are as yet developing. Ladies can also take a calcium supplement or a multivitamin.

Dairy items like milk, yogurt, and cheddar are great sources of calcium. Non-fat (skim) and low-fat dairy have equivalent measures of calcium and fewer calories than higher-fat dairy. Different sources of calcium include; dull green, verdant vegetables, dried beans and peas, nuts and seeds, and sardines.

Calcium-strengthened food varieties and refreshments are additionally great sources of calcium. These include orange juices, soy milk, tofu, almond milk, and breakfast cereals. It is most straightforward to meet your calcium needs through dairy food varieties. On the off chance that you are a veggie-lover, have lactose narrow-mindedness, or a milk sensitivity, ask your medical services supplier how to polish off sufficient calcium.

Pregnant ladies shouldn't polish off crude (unpasteurized) milk or eat food varieties that contain crude milk. Crude milk can expand the gamble of exceptionally hazardous foodborne sicknesses.

Vitamin D

Vitamin D is significant for calcium assimilation, insusceptible capability and cerebrum well-being. Daylight is one source of Vitamin D. Around five to ten minutes of daylight to bare arms or the face can supply a day of Vitamin D. These times can fluctuate contingent upon your topographical area and skin tone. Milk or yogurt with added Vitamin D can assist you with meeting your day-to-day needs. Slick fish, mushrooms, strengthened cereals, and dietary enhancements contain vitamin D.

Iron

Iron brings oxygen through the blood and conveys it all through the body. It additionally helps with insusceptibility, mental health, and digestion. Around 90% of the iron in the body is reused consistently. The developing child also stores sufficient iron to endure through the initial not many long stretches of life.
Pregnant ladies have an expanded measure of blood in their bodies, so they need more iron than non-pregnant ladies. Animal sources,

including red meat, fish, poultry, and eggs, are wealthy in iron. Different choices include enhanced and entire-grain bread, cereals, and pasta. Green verdant vegetables, beans, nuts, eggs, and dried organic products are reputable sources.

The iron found in animal sources differs from that found in plant sources. The body doesn't retain the iron in that frame of mind, nor the iron in meat, fish, and poultry. Be that as it may, iron retention can increment when eaten with food varieties high in L-ascorbic acid (like squeezed orange or red ringer peppers). An enrolled dietitian can suggest iron-rich food varieties and food varieties that can assist with iron ingestion. Numerous ladies enter pregnancy with low iron stores. Your medical services supplier might suggest iron supplementation at the principal pre-birth visit. A few ladies may likewise require evaluating for lack of iron on a continuous premise. Take iron enhancements between dinners, with water or squeeze, and not with different enhancements. Substances in espresso, tea, and milk can restrain iron assimilation. Taking iron enhancements at sleep time might assist with diminishing irritated stomach and additionally acid reflux.

Folic Corrosive/Folate/Vitamin B9

Folic corrosive, a B nutrient expected to assist the child with developing, is key previously and all through pregnancy. Folic corrosive diminishes spina bifida and other birth imperfections of the cerebrum and spinal string, called brain tube surrenders (NTDs). "Folate" is the term for the various types of supplements tracked down normally in food varieties. "Folic corrosive" is utilized in supplements and advanced grain items.

Improved bread, flour, pasta, rice, cereals, and other grain items are normal food wellsprings of folic corrosive. To check whether your food contains folic corrosive, check food names to check whether the food contains folic corrosive or folate.

There are numerous ways of meeting your folate/folic corrosive requirements. In the first place, take a multivitamin with folic corrosive. Additionally, ensure to eat bunches of foods grown from the ground, improved grain items,

vegetables (like peanuts), and organic citrus products.
A fluctuated, and adjusted veggie-lover diet should give you and your child adequate supplements during pregnancy.
You may find it more challenging to get sufficient iron and vitamin B12.
Converse with a maternity specialist or specialist about ensuring you're getting enough of these effective supplements.

Veggie lovers or vegetarian moms

Eating strongly during pregnancy is significant for your well-being and the soundness of your developing child.
It's essential to eat a fluctuated and adjusted diet during pregnancy to give you an adequate number of supplements and also aid the development of your child.
For the fact that you're pregnant and a veggie lover or vegetarian, you want to ensure you get sufficient iron, and vitamin B12, which are for the most part tracked down in meat and fish, and vitamin D, calcium and iodine.

Iron in your eating routine

Great sources of iron for veggie lovers and vegetarians include:

Beats

Dull green vegetables

The entire dinner was bread and flour

Nuts

Strengthened breakfast cereals (with added iron)

Dried natural products, like apricots

Vitamin B12 in your eating routine

Great sourcs of vitamin B12 for veggie lovers incorporate milk, cheddar and eggs.

Breakfast cereals are strengthened with vitamin B12.

Unsweetened soya drinks strengthened with vitamin B12

Yeast extricate, like Marmite, and nourishing yeast pieces which are strengthened with vitamin B12

Vitamin D in your eating routine

Although we get vitamin D from daylight, veggie lover food sources include:

Egg yolk
Food varieties strengthened with vitamin D, including a few breakfast bowls of cereal and fat spreads.
Dietary enhancements
Since vitamin D is found exclusively in a few food varieties, getting enough from varieties that normally contain vitamin D and strengthened food varieties alone is challenging.
You might be at a specific risk of not having sufficient vitamin D if:
You cover your skin when outside or invest bunches of energy inside.
You should consider taking a daily supplement of vitamin D throughout the year. Converse with a maternity specialist or specialist for exhortation.
If you're a veggie lover, look at the type of supplement to ensure your vitamin D is reasonable for vegetarians.

Calcium in your eating routine

For the fact that you're a veggie-lover, you need to ensure you get sufficient calcium. It is because non-veggie lovers get the most calcium from dairy food varieties.

Great sources of calcium for veggie lovers include:

Dull green verdant vegetables

Beats

Strengthened unsweetened soya, pea and oat drinks

Brown and white bread

Calcium-set tofu

Sesame seeds and tahini

Dried natural product

Converse with your maternity specialist or specialist about getting every one of the supplements you want for yourself and your child.

Iodine in your eating routine

Great sources of iodine for veggie lovers incorporate cow's milk, dairy items and eggs. Iodine can be tracked down in plant food varieties, such as cereals and grains. However, the levels fluctuate contingent on how much iodine is in the dirt where the plants are developed.

If you're a veggie lover, consider taking an iodine supplement or eating food varieties strengthened with iodine, for example, a few sorts of plant-based diets.

Chapter 3

Some food substances that could harm the growth and development of the baby

More food varieties can influence your well-being or your child's than you could understand. Figure out what food varieties to keep away from during pregnancy.

You need what's best for your child. That is why you add cut organic product to your strengthened breakfast cereal, top your servings of mixed greens with chickpeas and nibble on almonds. Be that as it may, do you know at least what food varieties to keep away from during pregnancy? Here's help figuring out pregnancy nourishment nuts and bolts.

Stay away from fish high in mercury: Fish can be an extraordinary wellspring of protein. The omega-3 unsaturated fats in many fish can advance your child's cerebrum and eye

improvement. Be that as it may, some fish and shellfish contain possibly hazardous degrees of mercury. An excessive amount of mercury could hurt your child's creating sensory system. The greater and more established the fish, the more mercury it will probably contain. During pregnancy, you are expected to stay away from:

- Bigeye fish
- Ruler mackerel
- Marlin
- Orange roughy
- Swordfish
- Shark
- Tilefish

So what what kind of fishes are better? A few kinds of fish contain little mercury.a few servings — of fish seven days during pregnancy. Consider:

- Anchovies
- Catfish
- Cod
- Herring
- Light canned fish
- Pacific shellfish
- Pollock
- Salmon

- Sardines
- Shad
- Shrimp
- Tilapia
- Trout

Be that as it may, limit white (tuna) fish.

Stay away from crude, half-cooked or polluted fish.

To stay away from destructive microorganisms or infections in fish:

- Keep away from crude fish and shellfish.

Instances of crude or half-cooked food varieties to keep away from incorporate sushi, sashimi, ceviche and crude shellfish, scallops or mollusks.

- Keep away from refrigerated, uncooked fish.

Models incorporate fish marked nova style, lox, kippered, smoked or jerky. Eating smoked fish on the off chance it's fixed in a goulash or other cooked dish is alright. Canned and rack-stable adaptations are additionally protected.

- Figure out neighborhood fish warnings. On the off chance that you eat fish from neighborhood waters, focus on nearby fish warnings — particularly on the off chance that water contamination is a worry. Assuming you are questionable about the well-being of fish you have proactively eaten, eat no other fish that week.

- Cook fish appropriately. Cook fish to an interior temperature of 145 F (63 C). Fish is done when it isolates into pieces and seems obscure all through. Cook shrimp, lobster and scallops until they're smooth white. Cook shellfishes, mussels and clams until their shells open. Dispose of any that don't open.

Stay away from half-cooked meat, poultry and eggs.

During pregnancy, you're at an expanded hazard of bacterial food contamination. Your response may be more extreme than if you weren't pregnant. Once in a long while, food contamination also influences the child.

To forestall foodborne sickness:

- Completely cook all meats and poultry before eating. Utilize a meat thermometer to ensure.
- Cook sausages and lunch get-together meats until they're steaming hot — or keep away from them. They can be wellsprings of an

interesting, however possibly serious foodborne sickness known as listeria contamination.

- Keep away from refrigerated pates and meat spreads. Canned and rack stable adaptations, be that as it may, are alright.
- Cook eggs until the egg yolks and whites are firm. Crude eggs can be polluted with destructive microscopic organisms.

Stay away from unpasteurized food varieties.

Some low-fat dairy items —skim milk, mozzarella cheddar and curds — can be a solid piece of your eating routine. Anything containing unpasteurized milk, be that as it may, is a no. These items could prompt foodborne sickness.

Avoid delicate cheeses, like brie, feta and blue cheddar, except if they are marked as being sanitized or made with purified milk. Additionally, try not to drink unpasteurized juice.

Keep away from unwashed products of the soil.

To dispense with destructive microscopic organisms:
Completely wash every crude food grown from the ground.
Stay away from crude fledglings of any sort — including horse feed, clover, radish and mung bean — which additionally could contain infection-causing microscopic organisms.
Make certain to cook sprouts completely.

Stay away from the overabundance of caffeine.
While caffeine can cross the placenta, the consequences for your child aren't clear.
Stay away from homegrown tea. There needs to be more information on the impacts of explicit spices on creating children. Subsequently, try not to drink homegrown tea except if your medical services supplier says it's alright —

Stay away from liquor.
No amount of liquor has been demonstrated to protect during pregnancy. The most secure bet is to stay away from liquor completely.

Think about the dangers. Drinking liquor during pregnancy prompts a higher gamble of an unnatural birth cycle and stillbirth. Drinking liquor may likewise bring about fetal liquor condition, which can cause facial disfigurements and loss of intellectual capacity. If you're worried about the liquor you drank before you realized you were pregnant or you assume you want assistance to quit drinking, seek counsel from your medicinal services supplier.

Chapter 4

Pregnancy stress and how to overcome it

What is Pre-birth Maternal Pressure?

Pre-birth maternal pressure alludes to the pressure that a mother encounters during her pregnancy.

Objective pressure alludes to how much difficulty a lady faces during a time of pressure. It can be estimated by the number of days she is presented to the stressor, the progressions that happen to her day-to-day existence, and the misfortunes she brings about because of the pressure (for example, cash or property). Emotional trouble alludes to a lady's very own response to the stressor. It can be estimated by evaluating her feelings and sentiments when presented with the distressing occasion.Pre-birth maternal pressure is very significant to take note of because most discoveries have found that the feeling of anxiety is related to negative outcomes in fetal and newborn child development.

When an individual is presented with an occasion seen as distressing, the cerebrum sets off an outpouring of occasions, eventually prompting the arrival of stress chemicals like cortisol. These pressure chemicals assist with setting up the person to adapt to the stressor. Notwithstanding, it has been exhibited that in pregnant ladies, these chemicals can pass from the mother to the baby through the placenta. This is upheld by studies that have found high maternal cortisol levels compared with high fetal cortisol levels. Openness to high cortisol levels can then present unfortunate results to the developing foetus.. Additionally, it has been exhibited that in utero, openness to high degrees of cortisol likewise influences post-natal events. In this manner, an essential objective of Twisting is to all the more likely figure out the impacts of intense and persistent pressure openness on youngster improvement, as well as the components by which maternal pressure acts to force these impacts.

Step-by-step instructions to conquer pressure and remain mentally collected during pregnancy

Numerous hopeful moms are in a condition of pressure during pregnancy. They don't have the foggiest idea of how to manage their feelings of trepidation and feelings. Some of the time, they feel the absence of consideration and correspondence. These straightforward strategies will assist pregnant ladies with remaining mentally collected and having a positive state of mind. Additionally, they are reasonable for everybody.

Stress during pregnancy is exceptionally hazardous for the soundness of ladies and children. All individuals are impacted by specific distressing variables consistently. Be that as it may, managing close-to-home pressure during pregnancy is difficult for future moms. Much here relies upon the endocrine profile state here.

How to conquer pressure and nervousness during pregnancy? Indeed, it is normal for some first opportunity to be mums. Here is this assist post to assist you with feeling delightful and quiet.

Here are straightforward yet successful ways of understanding how to manage pressure during pregnancy:

Envision Your Fantasies

For quite some time, the representation procedure has been recognizable to many individuals. The time has come to remember your growing-up experience and fantasize. To conquer pressure during early pregnancy, Walkthrough the moist sand or wet morning grass, pay attention to the sprinkling of the waves and the melody of the birds and take a gander at the beams of the sun getting through the thick foliage. Representation of wonderful minutes assists with limiting the impacts of pressure during pregnancy on baby and youngster advancement and dispose of mental and actual inconvenience. Coincidentally, this mental procedure will permit you to unwind during labour. Meanwhile, it will add to disposing of pressure during pregnancy and help to discover an authentic sense of reconciliation of psyche and adapt to restless encounters.

Breathe in Wonderful Fragrances to Conquer Pressure During Pregnancy

Fragrance-based treatment can be one more successful method for combatting pressure during late pregnancy. You can consolidate this strategy with different procedures. Before rehearsing unwinding or representation, air your room and fill it with the fragrance of any rejuvenating ointment that encourages you. You can blend a few oils simultaneously to upgrade the unwinding impact and battle pressure during pregnancy, all the more successfully. Bergamot and rose oil will diminish the psycho-close-to-home pressure. The fragrances of petitgrain have a great enemy of stress properties. Additionally, lavender oil will quiet you and help you adapt to a sleeping disorder and stress during pregnancy.

Speak with Cheerful Individuals

All the time, our current circumstance makes us blissful or despondent. Relationship stress during pregnancy emerges from challenges in speaking with individuals. Along these lines, talking with positive-disapproved individuals and breaking point of contact with those who debilitate you is essential. If something is irritating you, meeting with a hopeful companion is the best solution for stress during pregnancy. Don't hesitate to share your contemplations and fears for even a moment, since talking about them can diminish the power of pressure during pregnancy. Many investigations affirm that agreeable individuals conquer close-to-home encounters without any problem. Be that as it may, don't concentrate just on your concerns. Change to different subjects. For instance, check out the undertakings of your companion. It will likewise assist with diverting yourself from stress during pregnancy for some time.

Be Imaginative

Regardless of whether you view yourself as imaginative, you ought to attempt this technique. Take a stab at attracting or earth demonstrating to conquer side effects of pressure. Discharge your feelings.

Remember,the most exciting thing isn't the outcome but the innovative approach. Here is one more extraordinary method for disposing of pressure. This is an intuitive drawing. You needn't bother to be a craftsman by any stretch of the imagination. You could draw with your fingers, not with brushes. It advantageously affects the working of the sensory system. Trust your instinct, and it will let you know what to draw.

Invest More Energy Outside

This suggestion is particularly significant for women who experience pressure at work during pregnancy. Attempt to work less and invest more energy strolling outside. If you don't have the chance to leave town, go for a stroll in the city park. Try not to rush. Partake in the birdsong and delightful blossoms. Try not to contemplate the issues. Allow your body to turn into a solitary entire with nature. Focus on breathing to figure out how to conquer pressure during pregnancy. Breathe in however much clean air as could reasonably be expected being outside. Take full breaths and slow exhalations.

Try out some exercises

sports preparation is the best method for managing fears and close-to-home pressure. Running is the best solution for stress during pregnancy. Is it hard to run? You can move. Music and actual work make a twofold impact. The most exciting thing is to do something other than overburden yourself with working out. Along these lines, you can hurt yourself and your child. Focus on calm exercises that help you unwind, conquer pressure during pregnancy, and reinforce your body: attempt yoga or Pilates.

Recollect about Sound Nourishment

Hopeful moms frequently spoil themselves with desserts and permit themselves to eat low-quality food. Sometimes, they can't help suspecting that such items might assist with adapting to close-to-home pressure during pregnancy. The lack of nutrients and minerals prompts the consumption of the sensory system. Along these lines, a lady's body turns out to be significantly more defenceless against stress. Attempt to practice good eating habits and nutritious food varieties. Disregard consuming fewer calories for weight reduction; they can be exceptionally hazardous during this period. Eat more protein food varieties to get a ton of energy. Remember the advantages of foods grown from the ground. Drink newly pressed juices. For instance, pomegranate juice is a successful solution for stress during pregnancy. Disregard greasy, broiled, and salted dishes.

Conclusion

Congrats, as you have successfully gotten to the end of this book, and I trust it has fulfilled your inquiries on the right nourishments to take during pregnancy. I encourage you today to begin a sound practice and eat the best food varieties for your pregnancy to keep you and your child solid, and for you to prevail in this, make sure to avoid food varieties or substances that could hurt you and your child's turn of events and wellbeing like caffeine, liquor, cigarettes e.t.c. Additionally, note that anything you take in generally influences the child, so attempt however much as could reasonably be expected to eat sound foods, take the right nutrients and supplements and stay away from low-quality foods. With this expressed up until this point, never disregard water consumption since it will supplant each lost liquid from your body and prevent you from dehydrating. Water likewise plays a significant part in transporting these fundamental supplements around your body to where they are required. Continuously play it safe in any activity you participate in to try not to hurt the child's improvement and development.

www.ingramcontent.com/pod-product-compliance
Lightning Source LLC
LaVergne TN
LVHW020534160826
845677LV00015B/4059

9798368038513